5 – HTP FOR BEGINNERS

Harnessing Serotonin, Your Comprehensive Guide To Unlocking The Power Of 5-HTP For Mental Wellness, Stress Relief And Emotional Balance

Georgette Lockett

DISCLAIMER

The author of this book is not affiliated, associated, endorsed, sponsored, or approved by any company or individual. The views and opinions expressed in this book are solely those of the author and do not necessarily reflect the official policy or position of any entity.

The author hereby disclaims any relationship, collaboration, or partnership with any company or individual mentioned in this book. Any references to products, services, or individuals are provided for informational purposes only and should not be construed as an endorsement or recommendation.

Readers are advised to exercise their own judgment and discretion when applying the information provided in this book. The author shall not be held responsible for any actions taken by readers based on the content of this book.

This book is intended for general informational purposes only, and the author makes no representations or warranties of any kind, express or implied, about the completeness, accuracy, reliability, suitability, or availability of the information contained herein. Any reliance on the information in this book is at the reader's own risk.

The author reserves the right to update, change, or modify any information in this book without notice. It is the responsibility of the reader to verify any information before taking any actions based on the content of this book.

By reading this book, the reader acknowledges and agrees to the terms of this disclaimer.

Table of Contents

INTRODUCTION

5-HTP, or 5-Hydroxytryptophan, is a naturally occurring molecule that is essential for serotonin production in the human body. 5-HTP has attracted attention for its possible influence on mental health and general well-being as an intermediary in the manufacture of serotonin, a neurotransmitter typically connected with mood regulation. This chapter presents an overview of 5-HTP, diving into its history and emphasizing its importance in health promotion.

Overview Of 5-HTP

5-HTP is generated from tryptophan, an amino acid that is a precursor to serotonin. 5-HTP is found in a variety of plants and animals, but it is most typically derived from the seeds of the Griffonia simplicifolia plant. When 5-HTP is consumed, it passes the blood-brain barrier and is transformed into serotonin, which influences a variety of physiological activities such as mood, sleep, and hunger.

Historical Background

The origins of 5-HTP may be traced back to the mid-twentieth century when researchers started investigating its involvement in serotonin production. 5-HTP was first found as an intermediary chemical in the process from tryptophan to serotonin, but it quickly acquired attention in the scientific community due to its potential medicinal benefits. Its usage has expanded outside research facilities over the years to become a popular nutritional supplement.

Importance In Health And Well-Being

The importance of 5-HTP in health and well-being stems from its interaction with serotonin, a neurotransmitter that regulates mood and emotional equilibrium. Depression, anxiety, and sleeplessness have all been related to serotonin deficit. 5-HTP has been studied as a natural intervention to enhance mental health and emotional stability since it is a direct precursor to serotonin.

According to research, 5-HTP supplementation may lead to increased mood, less depressive symptoms, and better sleep quality. Given the effect of serotonin on satiety and food intake regulation, it has also been studied for its possible function in appetite control and weight management.

As with any dietary supplement, consumers should take 5-HTP with caution and under the supervision of a healthcare practitioner. Understanding the historical backdrop and the compound's importance in health and well-being lays the groundwork for making educated judgments about incorporating it into one's wellness regimen.

We will explore more into the mechanisms of action, possible advantages, and concerns related to 5-HTP supplementation in the next chapters. Investigating its effects on mental health, sleep, and other elements of well-being will give a thorough knowledge of the role 5-HTP plays in creating a better and more balanced lifestyle.

CHAPTER 1

Understanding 5-HTP

5-Hydroxytryptophan, or 5-HTP, is an important precursor of the neurotransmitter serotonin. It is derived from the amino acid tryptophan and plays an important role in a variety of physiological activities. Understanding 5-HTP entails investigating its origins, processes, and importance in human health.

What Is 5-HTP?

5-HTP is a naturally occurring molecule that the body produces from tryptophan, an important amino acid contained in dietary proteins. It is a critical building ingredient in the manufacture of serotonin, a neurotransmitter that regulates mood, sleep, and hunger. This chemical, which is marketed as a nutritional supplement, is commercially synthesized from the seeds of Griffonia simplicifolia, a West African shrub.

Sources And Production

Tryptophan is derived from dietary proteins such as meat, chicken, fish, dairy, nuts, and seeds. Inside the body, tryptophan goes through a sequence of enzymatic transformations to generate 5-HTP, which is subsequently converted into serotonin. The extraction of 5-HTP from Griffonia simplicifolia seeds is a meticulous procedure that results in a supplement form acceptable for ingestion.

Mechanism Of Action In The Body

After being ingested, 5-HTP passes the blood-brain barrier and enters the central nervous system, where it acts as a direct precursor of serotonin. Serotonin is well-known for its ability to regulate mood and promote emotions of well-being and satisfaction.

Serotonin also affects sleep patterns, eating regulation, and cognitive abilities. 5-HTP may benefit mental health, emotional balance, and general well-being by raising serotonin levels.

Recognizing 5-HTP's potential to regulate serotonin synthesis is key to understanding its mechanism in the body. Unlike tryptophan, which competes with other amino acids for transport across the blood-brain barrier, it avoids the rate-limiting phase in serotonin production. Because of its direct conversion into serotonin, 5-HTP is a viable supplement for illnesses associated with serotonin insufficiency.

The importance of 5-HTP in health and well-being stems from its possible medicinal uses. According to research, it may help with symptoms of sadness, anxiety, and sleeplessness. Furthermore, it has been studied for its involvement in migraine management, binge eating episodes reduction, and fibromyalgia symptom improvement.

5-HTP has historically received interest owing to its role in serotonin production and its therapeutic effects. Its popularity as a dietary supplement has expanded over time, as people seek natural options to enhance emotional balance and mental wellness.

As we learn more about 5-HTP, we see how it may be used to treat a variety of health issues. The entire study of 5-HTP provides insight into its considerable influence on general well-being, from its beginnings in the body's biochemical processes to its function as a precursor to serotonin.

CHAPTER 2

Role Of 5-HTP In Brain Health

5-HTP And Serotonin Production

5-Hydroxytryptophan (5-HTP) is important for brain health because of its interaction with serotonin, a neurotransmitter that is essential for mood regulation, sleep, and general emotional well-being. 5-HTP is a molecule derived from the amino acid tryptophan that acts as a precursor to the creation of serotonin in the brain.

5-HTP reaches the central nervous system after crossing the blood-brain barrier. A sequence of enzymatic processes involving aromatic L-amino acid decarboxylase converts it to serotonin. Serotonin, sometimes known as the "feel-good" neurotransmitter, has an impact on a variety of physiological and psychological activities.

Effects On Mood Regulation

5-HTP has a major influence on mood control. Depression, anxiety, and other mood problems have all been related to serotonin deficit. 5-HTP supplementation has shown potential in relieving symptoms linked with several illnesses by raising serotonin levels. According to research, regulating serotonin levels may improve mood by fostering emotions of well-being and satisfaction.

5-HTP has been studied for its ability to alleviate depression and anxiety symptoms. While additional study is needed, preliminary studies suggest that taking 5-HTP supplements may help those suffering from mild to severe depression and anxiety by regulating serotonin levels.

Impact On Mental Health Disorders

The importance of 5-HTP in mental health goes beyond mood disorders. Some studies have looked at its potential for treating disorders including sleeplessness, migraines, and fibromyalgia. 5-HTP may improve sleep patterns by modifying serotonin levels, as well as reduce the intensity and frequency of headaches and alleviate symptoms associated with fibromyalgia, a chronic pain disease.

However, it is critical to treat these results with caution. The effects of 5-HTP supplementation may differ from person to person, and its usage should be reviewed with a healthcare expert, particularly when treating specific mental health conditions or mixing it with other drugs.

Understanding the complex balance of neurotransmitters and their influence on mental health is a developing field of study. While 5-HTP shows promise in assisting with a variety of brain-related diseases by promoting serotonin synthesis, further research is needed to evaluate its effectiveness, ideal dose, and long-term consequences.

The ability of 5-HTP to favorably influence brain health emphasizes the significance of ongoing scientific research to efficiently harness its advantages while assuring its safe and responsible usage.

CHAPTER 3

5-HTP And Sleep

5-HTP, which is extracted from the seeds of the African plant Griffonia simplicifolia, has gotten a lot of interest for its possible role in encouraging good sleep patterns. Its impact on neurotransmitters in the brain, notably serotonin and melatonin, is inextricably tied to its association with sleep.

Influence On Sleep Patterns

Serotonin, a neurotransmitter generated from 5-HTP, is used by the body to make melatonin, a hormone important for regulating sleep-wake cycles. Melatonin signals to the body that it is time to sleep, and it is crucial in sustaining circadian rhythms.

5-HTP indirectly enhances melatonin production by boosting serotonin levels. This mechanism implies that taking 5-HTP supplements may help with sleep pattern regulation, perhaps decreasing the time it takes to fall asleep and enhancing overall sleep quality.

Role In Sleep Disorders

5-HTP has been studied for its potential utility in treating sleep problems such as insomnia. According to several research, 5-HTP supplementation may help improve sleep duration and quality in those who suffer from sleep disorders. Its capacity to increase serotonin levels, which encourages melatonin generation, may help to restore interrupted sleep patterns.

However, although the first results are encouraging, a more thorough study is required to get clear conclusions on the usefulness of 5-HTP in treating certain sleep problems.

Impact On Sleep Quality

Individual reactions to 5-HTP for sleep might differ. Some people may experience improvements in sleep latency (the time it takes to fall asleep) or total sleep length after taking 5-HTP supplements. Others may not have the same reactions.

The effect of 5-HTP on sleep may be influenced by factors such as dose, individual biochemistry, underlying health issues, and concomitant drugs. Furthermore, the usage of 5-HTP for sleep-related issues should be done with caution, ideally under the supervision of a healthcare practitioner.

In conclusion, although the association between 5-HTP and sleep seems promising, more extensive research is required to demonstrate its efficacy and safety profile, especially in the context of diverse sleep disorders. Its possible impact on serotonin and melatonin levels suggests an intriguing path for future study into non-pharmacological techniques to support good sleep patterns.

Individuals contemplating 5-HTP supplementation for sleep-related issues should speak with a healthcare physician to evaluate suitable doses, examine possible interactions with current drugs, and ensure a thorough grasp of the consequences of their unique situation.

CHAPTER 4

5-HTP And Weight Management

5-Hydroxytryptophan, or 5-HTP, has received attention for its possible involvement in weight loss. One significant area of investigation is how it affects appetite management and how it is believed to affect weight reduction attempts.

Appetite Regulation

5-HTP is required for the production of serotonin, a neurotransmitter involved in mood modulation and appetite control. Serotonin increases feelings of fullness and may aid in the suppression of cravings. 5-HTP may lead to lower hunger and consequent calorie intake by raising serotonin levels in the brain, thereby benefiting weight control.

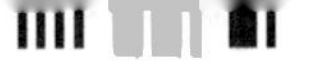

Impact On Weight Loss Efforts

5-HTP pills have been studied for their potential to aid in weight reduction. According to some studies, those who take 5-HTP tablets may have lower food intake and a sensation of fullness, resulting in lower calorie consumption. This might lead to a more controllable approach to weight reduction by lowering total food consumption.

Studies And Research Findings

Several research have been conducted to evaluate the effects of 5-HTP on weight control. While some studies have demonstrated promising outcomes in terms of hunger control and weight reduction, the findings aren't generally clear. The results are often variable owing to variables such as dose, individual variability, and research length.

Furthermore, the effect of 5-HTP on weight reduction may be more obvious in particular populations or under certain settings. Individuals with illnesses marked by disturbed satiety signals, for example, or those prone to emotional eating tendencies, may benefit more significantly from 5-HTP treatment.

While preliminary research suggests that 5-HTP may help people lose weight by suppressing their appetite, these results should be interpreted with care. Weight control is a multifaceted process driven by a variety of variables such as nutrition, activity, genetics, and general lifestyle.

In conclusion, 5-HTP seems to have a function in appetite control and may aid in weight loss attempts by affecting feelings of fullness and lowering food intake. More extensive and long-term trials, however, are required to confirm its usefulness and safety. Incorporating 5-HTP supplements into weight reduction programs should be done under the supervision of a healthcare practitioner, taking into account individual health circumstances and any potential drug interactions. As with any supplement, a well-balanced strategy that includes a nutritious diet and regular exercise is critical for effective and long-term weight control.

CHAPTER 5

5-HTP And Neurological Conditions

5-Hydroxytryptophan (5-HTP), a naturally occurring amino acid, has received interest for its function in mood modulation as well as its possible influence on neurological diseases. This chapter delves into the interesting link between 5-HTP and a variety of neurological illnesses.

Potential Benefits For Neurological Disorders

According to research, 5-HTP may have potential advantages for some neurological diseases. One important component is its capacity to pass the blood-brain barrier, which is essential for any chemical seeking to affect the central nervous system. 5-HTP may thereby alter the production of

The complicated nature of neurological illnesses, as well as the complex relationships inside the brain, need a thorough examination. 5-HTP research in the setting of Parkinson's disease, migraines, and other illnesses is promising but not yet definitive. As research advances, a more thorough knowledge of 5-HTP's involvement in brain health may emerge, opening up new treatment avenues.

CHAPTER 6

Safety And Side Effects Of 5-HTP

5-HTP, a precursor of serotonin, has received interest for its potential to treat mood disorders and other health issues. However, like with any supplement or medicine, understanding its safety profile, possible side effects, interactions, and recommended dose is critical for responsible usage.

Possible Adverse Effects

While 5-HTP is usually regarded as safe for most people when taken at authorized levels, it may produce moderate adverse effects in some people. These symptoms might include nausea, stomach discomfort, and diarrhea. In rare cases, people may develop headaches, dizziness, or tiredness.

Interactions And Precautions

Interactions with drugs or health problems are critical factors to consider. Antidepressants, notably selective serotonin reuptake inhibitors (SSRIs), monoamine oxidase inhibitors (MAOIs), and other drugs that influence serotonin levels, may interact with 5-HTP. Combining 5-HTP with certain medicines may result in serotonin syndrome, a potentially hazardous illness characterized by moderate to severe symptoms.

Individuals with pre-existing medical issues, such as cardiovascular illness or liver disease, as well as those who are pregnant or breastfeeding should seek the advice of a healthcare practitioner before taking 5-HTP. This cautious technique serves to limit possible dangers while also ensuring that it does not aggravate pre-existing conditions or interfere with current therapies.

Dosage Considerations

The proper dose of 5-HTP is critical for optimizing benefits while limiting dangers. Dosages might vary depending on individual requirements, health circumstances, and desired goals. Individual tolerance and effectiveness may be assessed by starting with lower dosages and progressively increasing them under physician supervision.

To avoid possible adverse effects, regular monitoring and adherence to appropriate doses are required. Furthermore, it's best to avoid suddenly discontinuing 5-HTP consumption, especially if you're taking it to treat mental health issues since this might cause withdrawal symptoms.

Understanding the 5-HTP safety profile is critical for prudent supplementation. While it has shown promise in improving mood and managing specific health concerns, its effects vary greatly across people. It is strongly advised to see a healthcare practitioner before beginning 5-HTP supplementation to guarantee its safe usage, particularly when taken with other drugs or in the presence of pre-existing health issues.

In conclusion, although 5-HTP has potential advantages for mood control and some health issues, it is critical to carefully assess its safety, possible side effects, interactions, and proper doses to successfully harness its good effects while minimizing any related dangers. Always make educated judgments and seek expert counsel for individualized recommendations and safe use.

CHAPTER 7

5-HTP And Pain Management

Influence On Pain Perception

5-HTP, a precursor of serotonin, has the potential to influence pain perception. Serotonin, which is often connected with mood control, also plays a function in pain signal modulation. According to research, changes in serotonin levels may have an influence on pain circuits within the neurological system. Serotonin receptors are found throughout the brain and spinal cord, where they influence pain signals and processing.

Fibromyalgia And 5-HTP

Fibromyalgia, a chronic condition marked by widespread musculoskeletal pain, exhaustion, and sleep difficulties, has piqued the attention of researchers studying 5-HTP.

According to some research, people with fibromyalgia may have low serotonin levels. Because 5-HTP is involved in serotonin production, it has been studied as a possible therapy for fibromyalgia symptoms. 5-HTP supplementation has been found to enhance pain intensity, sleep quality, and general well-being in some users, but larger-scale clinical research is required to confirm its effectiveness.

Other Pain-Related Conditions

In addition to fibromyalgia, 5-HTP has been studied in the treatment of various pain-related diseases such as headaches, migraines, and some neuropathic symptoms. Because of serotonin's role in pain regulation, researchers have been looking into whether changing serotonin levels with 5-HTP supplementation may help with certain disorders. While early study has shown encouraging results in lowering headache frequency and intensity, further research is needed to prove its efficacy and safety.

The function of 5-HTP in pain treatment is a growing topic of study and interest. Its effect on serotonin levels in the neurological system shows that it can modulate pain perception and improve symptoms in a variety of illnesses, including fibromyalgia and headaches. However, although the first results are encouraging, more solid clinical trials are required to verify its effectiveness, safety, and appropriate dose for various pain-related illnesses. Before beginning 5-HTP intake, as with any supplement or therapy, contact a healthcare expert, particularly if you have chronic pain.

CHAPTER 8

5-HTP And Stress Reduction

Stress has become a widespread problem in contemporary culture, affecting both mental health and general well-being. Understanding the function of 5-HTP in stress reduction gives insight into its potential usefulness in addressing this widespread problem.

Stress Response And 5-HTP

Hormones, neurotransmitters, and the nervous system all interact in intricate ways during the stress response. Serotonin, a neurotransmitter involved with mood control, is important to this reaction. As a precursor to serotonin, 5-HTP is essential. 5-HTP may influence stress reactions in the brain by raising serotonin levels, providing a calmer emotional state, and improving stress management.

Anxiety And Stress Management

Anxiety disorders, which are characterized by excessive concern and dread, often coexist with stress. According to research, serotonin depletion may lead to anxiety disorders. The capacity of 5-HTP to increase serotonin levels may reduce anxiety symptoms by generating a more balanced neurotransmitter environment. 5-HTP supplementation has demonstrated encouraging benefits in lowering anxiety symptoms, giving promise as an alternative approach to established therapy.

Role In Overall Well-Being

Chronic stress has a detrimental influence on overall well-being, impacting physical health, cognition, and emotional stability. 5-HTP supplementation may contribute to an increased feeling of well-being by modifying neurotransmitter levels, notably serotonin.

Elevating serotonin levels has been associated with decreased stress and anxiety, as well as improved sleep quality, improved mood, and higher resistance to stressors.

Considerations And Applications

While 5-HTP has the potential to reduce stress, its usage should be undertaken with caution. It is critical to understand individual requirements, dosage concerns, and possible pharmaceutical interactions. Before beginning 5-HTP supplementation, it is best to consult with a healthcare expert, particularly if you have a medical condition or are receiving treatment.

The interaction between stress, anxiety, and general well-being emphasizes the need for therapies such as 5-HTP. Its position as a precursor of serotonin suggests that it may be useful in the treatment of stress and anxiety disorders. Incorporating 5-HTP into a comprehensive stress management routine, along with healthy lifestyle choices, stress-relieving activities, and expert advice, may benefit an individual's mental and emotional health.

In conclusion, although 5-HTP has shown promise in stress reduction and anxiety management owing to its effect on serotonin levels, its usage should be carefully examined in combination with expert counsel and complete stress management measures for maximum benefits.

CHAPTER 9

Research And Clinical Studies

The excitement with 5-HTP derives from several research projects investigating its impact on human health. Several studies have been conducted to investigate its potential uses and effectiveness in treating a variety of illnesses.

Notable Research Findings

There has been a lot of research done on the impact of 5-HTP on mood disorders. Its significance in increasing serotonin levels, a neurotransmitter related to mood regulation, has been studied. Elevated serotonin levels have been related to enhanced mood and a possible decrease in sadness and anxiety symptoms. While many findings are encouraging, several studies have shown mixed or unclear outcomes in terms of effectiveness.

Furthermore, research into the effects of 5-HTP on sleep patterns has shown surprising results. Some studies show that 5-HTP may help regulate sleep cycles due to its impact on serotonin synthesis, thereby assisting patients with sleep difficulties.

Clinical Trials And Efficacy

Clinical investigations employing 5-HTP have given useful information. Researchers have investigated its significance in the treatment of disorders such as depression, anxiety, and fibromyalgia in controlled settings. While some studies have shown beneficial benefits, the findings vary, highlighting the need for further extensive study to reach conclusive conclusions.

Furthermore, exploratory research has looked into the possibility of 5-HTP in treating symptoms of neurological diseases such as Parkinson's disease. However, its usefulness as a stand-alone therapy is unknown and needs more research.

Future Prospects

5-HTP's potential medicinal uses continue to pique scientists' curiosity. Ongoing research is attempting to elucidate its mechanisms of action, optimal dosage, and potential synergies with other therapeutic interventions. Researchers are also investigating its potential significance in the treatment of stress-related diseases, chronic pain problems, and other neurological disorders.

However, difficulties remain in completely comprehending the complex. Further research is needed to clarify its long-term safety profile, identify certain subgroups that may benefit the most from its use, and refine its use instructions.

While current research emphasizes promising characteristics of 5-HTP, more extensive clinical trials are required to establish its effectiveness, safety, and broad application across a wide range of health issues.

In conclusion, current research on 5-HTP offers a possible path for treating specific health issues, notably those related to mood management, sleep disorders, and perhaps neurological diseases. However, more study is required to realize its full potential and develop precise criteria for its safe and effective usage.

CHAPTER 10

Integrating 5-HTP Into Daily Life

5-HTP, derived from Griffonia simplicifolia seeds, has received attention for its potential benefits on mood, sleep, and overall well-being. Incorporating 5-HTP into daily life involves understanding its uses, supplement considerations, and supportive lifestyle changes for maximum advantage.

Practical Applications

When considering 5-HTP supplementation, it's crucial to consult a healthcare provider. Dosage recommendations vary based on individual needs and health conditions. Typically, starting with lower doses and gradually increasing is advisable. Regular intake, usually divided throughout the day, ensures sustained effects.

For mood support, 5-HTP may be integrated as part of a holistic approach that includes stress management techniques, regular exercise, and a balanced diet rich in essential nutrients. However, it's essential to avoid combining 5-HTP with other serotonin-affecting medications without medical advice to prevent potential interactions.

Supplement Considerations

Selecting a reputable brand offering high-quality 5-HTP supplements is paramount. Look for products that undergo third-party testing to ensure purity, potency, and absence of contaminants. Considering the form of the supplement—capsules, tablets, or liquid—depends on personal preferences and ease of use.

Understanding the supplement's purity and dosage strength aids in making informed decisions. Some supplements may include additional ingredients, such as B vitamins or herbal extracts, intended to enhance their effects. Evaluating these additives and their potential benefits or interactions is advisable.

Lifestyle Changes For Maximum Benefit

While 5-HTP can offer support, combining it with lifestyle changes can amplify its positive effects. Regular exercise stimulates serotonin production, synergizing with 5-HTP's mechanisms. Additionally, maintaining a well-balanced diet, rich in whole grains, fruits, and vegetables, supports overall mental health.

Prioritizing quality sleep contributes significantly to emotional well-being. Establishing a consistent sleep schedule, creating a relaxing bedtime routine, and minimizing screen time before sleep can improve sleep quality, potentially complementing the effects of 5-HTP on sleep regulation.

Mindfulness practices, such as meditation or yoga, assist in stress reduction, working synergistically with 5-HTP's potential to support mood and stress management.

Incorporating 5-HTP into daily life isn't solely about supplementation; it's about adopting a holistic approach to well-being. While 5-HTP can provide support, its benefits are most profound when combined with healthy habits and a balanced lifestyle.

Understanding individual responses and consulting healthcare professionals to tailor supplementation, along with lifestyle modifications, is key to optimizing the benefits of 5-HTP and promoting overall mental and emotional wellness.

Conclusion

In summarizing the exploration into 5-HTP (5-Hydroxytryptophan), it becomes evident that this compound holds substantial promise in the realm of health and well-being. Throughout this comprehensive investigation, we've delved into its fundamental aspects, various roles, potential benefits, and safety considerations, painting a holistic picture of its impact.

Summary Of Key Points

The journey through 5-HTP has illuminated its origins, mechanisms of action and fundamental influence on brain health. We've discovered how it acts as a precursor to serotonin, impacting mood regulation, and mental health disorders, and potentially extending its effects to neurological conditions. Discussions highlighted its role in stress reduction, pain management, and its potential to enhance overall well-being.

Potential Future Developments

As research on 5-HTP advances, its promising applications continue to attract attention. Ongoing studies explore its efficacy in diverse domains, hinting at its potential role in addressing a wider array of health concerns.

The evolving understanding of 5-HTP's mechanisms and interactions opens doors for more targeted therapeutic interventions.

The significance of 5-HTP in health and well-being cannot be overstated. Its ability to modulate neurotransmitter function, particularly in the case of serotonin, underscores its relevance in mental health and emotional stability. Moreover, its potential in managing various health conditions, coupled with its relatively favorable safety profile, makes it a subject of keen interest among researchers and health enthusiasts alike.

While 5-HTP offers promise, it's essential to approach its utilization with an informed perspective. Caution and consultation with healthcare professionals remain crucial, especially when considering supplementation. Incorporating 5-HTP into daily routines must be balanced with lifestyle adjustments and comprehensive health management.

In conclusion, 5-HTP represents a fascinating avenue in the pursuit of holistic health. Its multifaceted roles in brain health, stress management, pain perception, and more paint a compelling picture of its potential contributions. As our understanding grows and research advances, 5-HTP stands as an intriguing area for further exploration and potential therapeutic applications.

THE END

55